Pocket Clinical Guide for

RADIOGRAPHIC IMAGE PRODUCTION AND MANIPULATION

Craig T. Shephard, MS, RT(R), RDMS

Program Director
School of Radiologic Technology
Metropolitan Nashville General Hospital
Nashville, Tennessee

D1235353

McGraw-Hill
MEDICAL PUBLISHING DIVISION

New York   Chicago   San Francisco   Lisbon   London   Madrid   Mexico City
Milan   New Delhi   San Juan   Seoul   Singapore   Sydney   Toronto

Pocket Clinical Guide for
Radiographic Image Production and Manipulation

4567890 WCT WCT 0987

Set ISBN 0-07-137577-5
Pocket Clinical Guide ISBN 0-07-141003-1
Book ISBN 0-07-141002-3

This book was set in Palatino by North Market Street Graphics.
The editors were Julie Scardiglia, Susan R. Noujaim, and Karen W. Davis.
The production supervisor was Catherine H. Saggese.

Quebecor/Taunton was printer and binder.

This book is printed on acid-free paper.

Contents

INTRODUCTION

This pocket clinical guide provides radiography students with a convenient reference to radiographic techniques and technical conversions used in the clinical setting. It includes several pages of blank technique charts that can be customized to one or more clinical affiliate sites by recording diagnostic exposure factors for each anatomical part. Students are encouraged to use a pencil when recording exposure factors, because these factors may need to be changed at some time during the program.

This guide highlights pertinent technical conversions and tips for altering exposure factors in various clinical situations. Radiographs demonstrating image quality accompany technical conversion information. The appendices provide tables listing information in a convenient format for quick reference. For more complete information pertaining to radiographic image production and technical conversions, refer to the accompanying *Radiographic Image Production and Manipulation* textbook.

Radiography students are encouraged to read the clinical guide to become familiar with its layout before using it in the clinical setting. The table of contents can also be used to find pertinent information.

2

Sample Technique Chart

Clinical Site: <u>Medical Center North</u>
**Room no. 10</u>

Anatomical part	Projection	Part thickness (cm)	mA	time(s)	mAs	kVp	SID (in.)	Cassette size (in.)/ placement	Speed (RS)	Grid ratio	AEC detector(s)	Conventional radiography (✓)	CR (✓)	DR (✓)
Hip	AP	20	200	.2	40	75	40	10 x 12 LW	250	12:1	☐ ■ ☐	✓		
											☐ ☐ ☐			
											☐ ☐ ☐			
											☐ ☐ ☐			
											☐ ☐ ☐			
											☐ ☐ ☐			

CLASSIFICATION: _____

Clinical Site: _____
Room no. _____

Anatomical part	Projection	Part thickness (cm)	mA	time(s)	mAs	kVp	SID (in.)	Cassette size (in.)/ placement	Speed (RS)	Grid ratio	AEC detector(s)	Conventional radiography (✓)	CR (✓)	DR (✓)
											☐ ☐ ☐			
											☐ ☐ ☐			
											☐ ☐ ☐			
											☐ ☐ ☐			
											☐ ☐ ☐			
											☐ ☐ ☐			
											☐ ☐ ☐			
											☐ ☐ ☐			
											☐ ☐ ☐			
											☐ ☐ ☐			

CLASSIFICATION: _____

3

Clinical Site: _____

Room no. _____

Anatomical part	Projection	Part thickness (cm)	mA	time(s)	mAs	kVp	SID (in.)	Cassette size (in.)/ placement	Speed (RS)	Grid ratio	AEC detector(s)	Conventional radiography (✓)	CR (✓)	DR (✓)
											☐ ☐ ☐			
											☐ ☐ ☐			
											☐ ☐ ☐			
											☐ ☐ ☐			
											☐ ☐ ☐			
											☐ ☐ ☐			
											☐ ☐ ☐			
											☐ ☐ ☐			
											☐ ☐ ☐			
											☐ ☐ ☐			

CLASSIFICATION: _____

Clinical Site: _____
Room no. _____

Anatomical part	Projection	Part thickness (cm)	mA	time(s)	mAs	kVp	SID (in.)	Cassette size (in.)/ placement	Speed (RS)	Grid ratio	AEC detector(s)	Conventional radiography (✓)	CR (✓)	DR (✓)
											☐ ☐ ☐			
											☐ ☐ ☐			
											☐ ☐ ☐			
											☐ ☐ ☐			
											☐ ☐ ☐			
											☐ ☐ ☐			
											☐ ☐ ☐			
											☐ ☐ ☐			
											☐ ☐ ☐			
											☐ ☐ ☐			

CLASSIFICATION: _____

Clinical Site: _____
Room no. _____

Anatomical part	Projection	Part thickness (cm)	mA	time(s)	mAs	kVp	SID (in.)	Cassette size (in.)/placement	Speed (RS)	Grid ratio	AEC detector(s)	Conventional radiography (✓)	CR (✓)	DR (✓)
											☐ ☐ ☐			
											☐ ☐ ☐			
											☐ ☐ ☐			
											☐ ☐ ☐			
											☐ ☐ ☐			
											☐ ☐ ☐			
											☐ ☐ ☐			
											☐ ☐ ☐			
											☐ ☐ ☐			

CLASSIFICATION: _____

Clinical Site: _____

Room no. _____

Anatomical part	Projection	Part thickness (cm)	mA time(s)	mAs	kVp	SID (in.)	Cassette size (in.)/ placement	Speed (RS)	Grid ratio	AEC detector(s)	Conventional radiography (✓)	CR (✓)	DR (✓)
										☐☐☐			
										☐☐☐			
										☐☐☐			
										☐☐☐			
										☐☐☐			
										☐☐☐			
										☐☐☐			
										☐☐☐			
										☐☐☐			

CLASSIFICATION: _____

7

8

Clinical Site: _____
Room no. _____

Anatomical part	Projection	Part thickness (cm)	mA / time(s)	mAs	kVp	SID (in.)	Cassette size (in.)/ placement	Speed (RS)	Grid ratio	AEC detector(s)	Conventional radiography (✓)	CR (✓)	DR (✓)
										☐ ☐ ☐			
										☐ ☐ ☐			
										☐ ☐ ☐			
										☐ ☐ ☐			
										☐ ☐ ☐			
										☐ ☐ ☐			
										☐ ☐ ☐			
										☐ ☐ ☐			
										☐ ☐ ☐			

CLASSIFICATION: _____

Clinical Site: _____

Room no. _____

Anatomical part	Projection	Part thickness (cm)	mA time(s)	mAs	kVp	SID (in.)	Cassette size (in.)/ placement	Speed (RS)	Grid ratio	AEC detector(s)	Conventional radiography (✓)	CR (✓)	DR (✓)
										☐☐☐			
										☐☐☐			
										☐☐☐			
										☐☐☐			
										☐☐☐			
										☐☐☐			
										☐☐☐			
										☐☐☐			
										☐☐☐			

CLASSIFICATION: _____

9

Clinical Site: _____
Room no. _____

Anatomical part	Projection	Part thickness (cm)	mA	time(s)	mAs	kVp	SID (in.)	Cassette size (in.)/ placement	Speed (RS)	Grid ratio	AEC detector(s)	Conventional radiography (✓)	CR (✓)	DR (✓)
											☐ ☐ ☐			
											☐			
											☐ ☐ ☐			
											☐			
											☐ ☐ ☐			
											☐			
											☐ ☐ ☐			
											☐			
											☐ ☐ ☐			
											☐			
											☐ ☐ ☐			
											☐ ☐			

CLASSIFICATION: _____

Clinical Site: _____
Room no. _____

Anatomical part	Projection	Part thickness (cm)	mA	time(s)	mAs	kVp	SID (in.)	Cassette size (in.)/ placement	Speed (RS)	Grid ratio	AEC detector(s)	Conventional radiography (✔)	CR (✔)	DR (✔)

CLASSIFICATION: _____

11

Clinical Site: _____

Room no. _____

Anatomical part	Projection	Part thickness (cm)	mA / time(s)	mAs	kVp	SID (in.)	Cassette size (in.)/ placement	Speed (RS)	Grid ratio	AEC detector(s)	Conventional radiography (✓)	CR (✓)	DR (✓)
										☐ ☐ ☐			
										☐ ☐ ☐			
										☐ ☐ ☐			
										☐ ☐ ☐			
										☐ ☐ ☐			
										☐ ☐ ☐			
										☐ ☐ ☐			
										☐ ☐ ☐			
										☐ ☐ ☐			
										☐ ☐ ☐			

CLASSIFICATION: _____

Clinical Site: _____

Room no. _____

Anatomical part	Projection	Part thickness (cm)	mA	time(s)	mAs	kVp	SID (in.)	Cassette size (in.)/ placement	Speed (RS)	Grid ratio	AEC detector(s)	Conventional radiography (✓)	CR (✓)	DR (✓)
											☐ ☐ ☐			
											☐ ☐ ☐			
											☐ ☐ ☐			
											☐ ☐ ☐			
											☐ ☐ ☐			
											☐ ☐ ☐			
											☐ ☐ ☐			
											☐ ☐ ☐			
											☐ ☐ ☐			

CLASSIFICATION: _____

13

Clinical Site: _____

Room no. _____

Anatomical part	Projection	Part thickness (cm)	mA time(s)	mAs	kVp	SID (in.)	Cassette size (in.)/ placement	Speed (RS)	Grid ratio	AEC detector(s)	Conventional radiography (✓)	CR (✓)	DR (✓)
										☐ ☐ ☐			
										☐ ☐			
										☐ ☐ ☐			
										☐ ☐			
										☐ ☐ ☐			
										☐ ☐			
										☐ ☐ ☐			
										☐ ☐			
										☐ ☐ ☐			
										☐ ☐			

CLASSIFICATION: _____

Clinical Site: _____

Room no. _____

Anatomical part	Projection	Part thickness (cm)	mA	time(s)	mAs	kVp	SID (in.)	Cassette size (in.)/ placement	Speed (RS)	Grid ratio	AEC detector(s)	Conventional radiography (✓)	CR (✓)	DR (✓)
											☐ ☐ ☐			
											☐ ☐ ☐			
											☐ ☐ ☐			
											☐ ☐ ☐			
											☐ ☐ ☐			
											☐ ☐ ☐			
											☐ ☐ ☐			
											☐ ☐ ☐			
											☐ ☐ ☐			
											☐ ☐ ☐			

CLASSIFICATION: _____

Clinical Site: _____

Room no. _____

Anatomical part	Projection	Part thickness (cm)	mA time(s)	mAs	kVp	SID (in.)	Cassette size (in.)/ placement	Speed (RS)	Grid ratio	AEC detector(s)	Conventional radiography (✓)	CR (✓)	DR (✓)
										☐ ☐ ☐			
										☐ ☐ ☐			
										☐ ☐ ☐			
										☐ ☐ ☐			
										☐ ☐ ☐			
										☐ ☐ ☐			
										☐ ☐ ☐			
										☐ ☐ ☐			
										☐ ☐ ☐			
										☐ ☐ ☐			

CLASSIFICATION: _____

Clinical Site: _____

Room no. _____

Anatomical part	Projection	Part thickness (cm)	mA	time(s)	mAs	kVp	SID (in.)	Cassette size (in.)/ placement	Speed (RS)	Grid ratio	AEC detector(s)	Conventional radiography (✓)	CR (✓)	DR (✓)
											☐☐☐			
											☐☐☐			
											☐☐☐			
											☐☐☐			
											☐☐☐			
											☐☐☐			
											☐☐☐			
											☐☐☐			
											☐☐☐			
											☐☐☐			

CLASSIFICATION: _____

Clinical Site: _____

Room no. _____

Anatomical part	Projection	Part thickness (cm)	mA	time(s)	mAs	kVp	SID (in.)	Cassette size (in.)/ placement	Speed (RS)	Grid ratio	AEC detector(s)	Conventional radiography (✓)	CR (✓)	DR (✓)
											☐ ☐ ☐			
											☐ ☐			
											☐ ☐			
											☐ ☐			
											☐ ☐			
											☐ ☐			
											☐ ☐			
											☐ ☐			
											☐ ☐ ☐			
											☐			

CLASSIFICATION: _____

Clinical Site: _____

Room no. _____

Anatomical part	Projection	Part thickness (cm)	mA	time(s)	mAs	kVp	SID (in.)	Cassette size (in.)/ placement	Speed (RS)	Grid ratio	AEC detector(s)	Conventional radiography (✓)	CR (✓)	DR (✓)
											☐☐☐			
											☐☐☐			
											☐☐☐			
											☐☐☐			
											☐☐☐			
											☐☐☐			
											☐☐☐			
											☐☐☐			
											☐☐☐			
											☐☐☐			

CLASSIFICATION: _____

Clinical Site: _____

Room no. _____

Anatomical part	Projection	Part thickness (cm)	mA / time(s)	mAs	kVp	SID (in.)	Cassette size (in.)/ placement	Speed (RS)	Grid ratio	AEC detector(s)	Conventional radiography (✓)	CR (✓)	DR (✓)
										☐ ☐ ☐			
										☐ ☐ ☐			
										☐ ☐ ☐			
										☐ ☐ ☐			
										☐ ☐ ☐			
										☐ ☐ ☐			
										☐ ☐ ☐			
										☐ ☐ ☐			
										☐ ☐ ☐			
										☐ ☐ ☐			

CLASSIFICATION: _____

Clinical Site: _____

Room no. _____

Anatomical part	Projection	Part thickness (cm)	mA	time(s)	mAs	kVp	SID (in.)	Cassette size (in.)/ placement	Speed (RS)	Grid ratio	AEC detector(s)	Conventional radiography (✓)	CR (✓)	DR (✓)
											☐ ☐ ☐			
											☐ ☐ ☐			
											☐ ☐ ☐			
											☐ ☐ ☐			
											☐ ☐ ☐			
											☐ ☐ ☐			
											☐ ☐ ☐			
											☐ ☐ ☐			
											☐ ☐ ☐			

CLASSIFICATION: _____

Clinical Site: _____

Room no. _____

Anatomical part	Projection	Part thickness (cm)	mA	time(s)	mAs	kVp	SID (in.)	Cassette size (in.)/ placement	Speed (RS)	Grid ratio	AEC detector(s)	Conventional radiography (✓)	CR (✓)	DR (✓)
											☐ ☐ ☐			
											☐ ☐ ☐			
											☐ ☐ ☐			
											☐ ☐ ☐			
											☐ ☐ ☐			
											☐ ☐ ☐			
											☐ ☐ ☐			
											☐ ☐ ☐			
											☐ ☐ ☐			

CLASSIFICATION: _____

Clinical Site: _____

Room no. _____

Anatomical part	Projection	Part thickness (cm)	mA time(s)		mAs	kVp	SID (in.)	Cassette size (in.)/ placement	Speed (RS)	Grid ratio	AEC detector(s)	Conventional radiography (✓)	CR (✓)	DR (✓)

CLASSIFICATION: _____

23

Clinical Site: _____

Room no. _____

24

Anatomical part	Projection	Part thickness (cm)	mA	time(s)	mAs	kVp	SID (in.)	Cassette size (in.)/ placement	Speed (RS)	Grid ratio	AEC detector(s)	Conventional radiography (✓)	CR (✓)	DR (✓)
											☐ ☐ ☐			
											☐ ☐ ☐			
											☐ ☐ ☐			
											☐ ☐ ☐			
											☐ ☐ ☐			
											☐ ☐ ☐			
											☐ ☐ ☐			
											☐ ☐ ☐			
											☐ ☐ ☐			

CLASSIFICATION: _____

Clinical Site: _____
Room no. _____

Anatomical part	Projection	Part thickness (cm)	mA | time(s)	mAs	kVp	SID (in.)	Cassette size (in.)/ placement	Speed (RS)	Grid ratio	AEC detector(s)	Conventional radiography (✓)	CR (✓)	DR (✓)
										▢ ▢ ▢			
										▢ ▢ ▢			
										▢ ▢ ▢			
										▢ ▢ ▢			
										▢ ▢ ▢			
										▢ ▢ ▢			
										▢ ▢ ▢			
										▢ ▢ ▢			
										▢ ▢ ▢			
										▢ ▢ ▢			

CLASSIFICATION: _____

Clinical Site: _____

Room no. _____

Anatomical part	Projection	Part thickness (cm)	mA / time(s)	mAs	kVp	SID (in.)	Cassette size (in.)/ placement	Speed (RS)	Grid ratio	AEC detector(s)	Conventional radiography (✓)	CR (✓)	DR (✓)
										☐ ☐ ☐			
										☐ ☐ ☐			
										☐ ☐ ☐			
										☐ ☐ ☐			
										☐ ☐ ☐			
										☐ ☐ ☐			
										☐ ☐ ☐			
										☐ ☐ ☐			
										☐ ☐ ☐			

CLASSIFICATION: _____

Clinical Site: _____

Room no. _____

Anatomical part	Projection	Part thickness (cm)	mA	time(s)	mAs	kVp	SID (in.)	Cassette size (in.)/ placement	Speed (RS)	Grid ratio	AEC detector(s)	Conventional radiography (✓)	CR (✓)	DR (✓)
											☐ ☐ ☐			
											☐			
											☐ ☐ ☐			
											☐			
											☐ ☐ ☐			
											☐			
											☐ ☐ ☐			
											☐			
											☐ ☐ ☐			
											☐			

CLASSIFICATION: _____

Clinical Site: _____

Room no. _____

Anatomical part	Projection	Part thickness (cm)	mA / time(s)	mAs	kVp	SID (in.)	Cassette size (in.)/ placement	Speed (RS)	Grid ratio	AEC detector(s)	Conventional radiography (✓)	CR (✓)	DR (✓)
										☐☐☐			
										☐☐☐			
										☐☐☐			
										☐☐☐			
										☐☐☐			
										☐☐☐			
										☐☐☐			
										☐☐☐			
										☐☐☐			

CLASSIFICATION: _____

Clinical Site: _____

Room no. _____

Anatomical part	Projection	Part thickness (cm)	mA	time(s)	mAs	kVp	SID (in.)	Cassette size (in.)/ placement	Speed (RS)	Grid ratio	AEC detector(s)	Conventional radiography (✓)	CR (✓)	DR (✓)
											☐☐☐			
											☐☐☐			
											☐☐☐			
											☐☐☐			
											☐☐☐			
											☐☐☐			
											☐☐☐			
											☐☐☐			
											☐☐☐			
											☐☐☐			

CLASSIFICATION: _____

Clinical Site: _____

Room no. _____

Anatomical part	Projection	Part thickness (cm)	mA / time(s)		mAs	kVp	SID (in.)	Cassette size (in.)/ placement	Speed (RS)	Grid ratio	AEC detector(s)	Conventional radiography (✓)	CR (✓)	DR (✓)

CLASSIFICATION: _____

Clinical Site: _____

Room no. _____

Anatomical part	Projection	Part thickness (cm)	mA / time(s)	mAs	kVp	SID (in.)	Cassette size (in.)/ placement	Speed (RS)	Grid ratio	AEC detector(s)	Conventional radiography (✓)	CR (✓)	DR (✓)
										☐ ☐ ☐			
										☐ ☐			
										☐ ☐ ☐			
										☐ ☐			
										☐ ☐ ☐			
										☐ ☐			
										☐ ☐ ☐			
										☐ ☐			
										☐ ☐ ☐			
										☐ ☐			

CLASSIFICATION: _____

TECHNICAL CONVERSIONS AFFECTING RADIOGRAPHIC DENSITY

When evaluating a film for proper density, you should first determine if the anatomical part or parts of interest are adequately penetrated. This applies to underexposure only, because a radiograph cannot be overexposed unless there is first sufficient penetration of the part. On an underexposed radiograph, you can determine if there is sufficient penetration by looking for structures that lie behind other structures (Fig. 1). If there is sufficient penetration, you should only

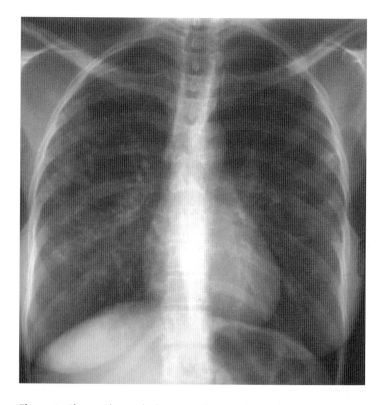

Figure 1 Chest radiograph demonstrating good x-ray beam penetration through the heart. Note the thoracic vertebrae and their interspaces, which indicate proper penetration through the heart. (Reproduced, with permission, from Slone RM, Guitierrez FR, Fisher AJ: *Thoracic Imaging.* McGraw-Hill, New York, 1999)

change the milliampere-seconds (mAs) setting to change density. If there is insufficient penetration and the radiograph is too light, you should only change the kilovoltage (kV) setting to increase both penetration and density. Therefore, it is important to only change one factor when changing density.

Overexposure and Underexposure

Generally, overexposure and underexposure are expressed as either 50% or 100% overexposed (dark) or underexposed (light) as follows:

- A little light = 50% light
- A little dark = 50% dark
- Very light = 100% light
- Very dark = 100% dark

> **Technical Tip:** Unless a radiograph is at least 50% too light or too dark, it is not necessary to repeat it to change density.

Milliampere-Seconds (mAs) Setting

> Refer to **Appendix A** for Milliampere-Seconds (mAs) Table

- **Radiograph is 50% light.** If you determine that a radiograph is 50% too light (and there is good penetration), you must increase the mAs by 50%. This is achieved by multiplying the mAs by 1.5. Figure 2 shows a radiograph that is 50% too light and the repeated radiograph made with the appropriate change in mAs.
- **Radiograph is 50% dark.** If you determine that a radiograph is 50% too dark, you must decrease the mAs by 25%. This is accomplished by multiplying the mAs by 0.75. Figure 3 shows a radiograph that is 50% too dark and the repeated radiograph made with the appropriate change in mAs.
- **Radiograph is 100% light.** If you determine a radiograph to be 100% too light (and there is good penetration), you must increase the mAs by 100%. This is accomplished by multiplying the mAs by 2.0. Figure 4 shows a radiograph that is 100% too light and the repeated radiograph made with the appropriate increase in mAs.

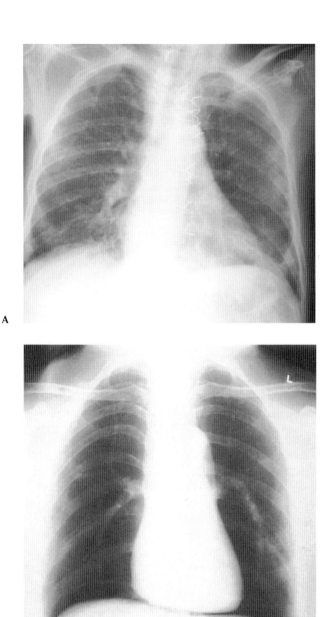

Figure 2 Comparison of (A) a 50% underexposed (light) chest radiograph with (B) a properly exposed chest radiograph. (*A* is reproduced, with permission, from Slone RM, Guitierrez FR, Fisher AJ: *Thoracic Imaging.* McGraw-Hill, New York, 1999; *B* from Saia DA: *Appleton & Lange's Review for the Radiography Examination,* 4th ed. McGraw-Hill, New York, 2000)

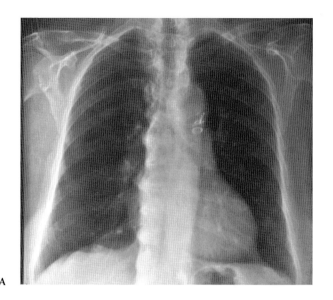

A

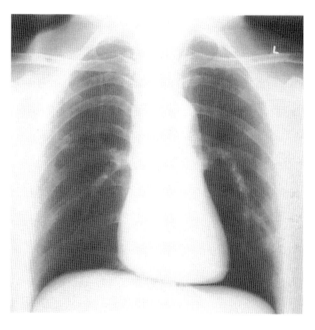

B

Figure 3 Comparison of (A) 50% overexposed (dark) chest radiograph with (B) a properly exposed chest radiograph. (*A* is reproduced, with permission, from Slone RM, Guitierrez FR, Fisher AJ: *Thoracic Imaging.* McGraw-Hill, New York, 1999; *B* from Saia DA: *Appleton & Lange's Review for the Radiography Examination,* 4th ed. McGraw-Hill, New York, 2000)

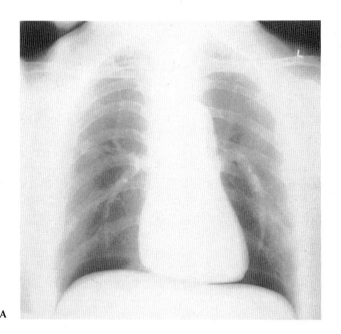

A

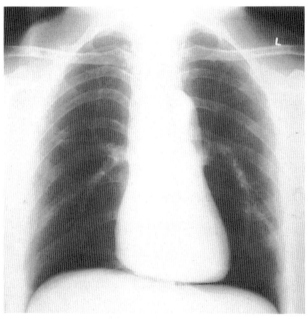

B

Figure 4 Comparison of (A) a 100% underexposed (light) chest radiograph with (B) a properly exposed chest radiograph. (Reproduced, with permission, from Saia DA: *Appleton & Lange's Review for the Radiography Examination,* 4th ed. McGraw-Hill, New York, 2000)

- **Radiograph is 100% dark.** If you determine a radiograph to be 100% too dark, you must decrease the mAs by 50%. This is accomplished by multiplying the mAs by 0.5. Figure 5 shows a radiograph that is 100% too dark and the repeated radiograph made with the appropriate decrease in mAs.

Technical Tip: It is difficult to determine the percentage of underexposure or overexposure on a severely underexposed or overexposed radiograph (over 100% light or dark). Radiographic density errors exceeding 100% should be rare, particularly if a technique chart is used. Therefore, if a radiograph is determined to be more than 100% too light or dark, first check the control panel to see if the wrong mAs setting was accidentally selected.

Kilovoltage Setting

Kilovoltage (kV) is a photographic factor that can be used to change both radiographic contrast and radiographic density. Changes in kV setting used to alter radiographic density also change radiographic contrast. A decrease in kV in order to decrease radiographic density can result in underpenetration of the anatomical part. You should therefore change the mAs setting to make radiographic density changes, unless you determine that the anatomical part is underpenetrated. If proper penetration exists, only the mAs setting should be adjusted to change radiographic density.

Changes in kV to alter density are governed by the *15% rule.* The **15% rule** states that a 15% kV increase produces a 100% density increase. A 15% kV decrease produces a 100% density decrease. Therefore, a 15% kV increase will have the same effect as doubling the mAs. Conversely, a 15% kV decrease will have the same effect as halving the mAs. The kV must be multiplied by 1.15 to increase it by 15%, whereas the kV must be multiplied by 0.85 to decrease it by 15%.

Technical Tip: Most technical conversions made to alter radiographic density should be accomplished by changing the mAs setting (assuming there is adequate penetration). Changes in kilovoltage settings should be reserved for altering radiographic contrast and for increasing radiographic density when the anatomical part is underpenetrated.

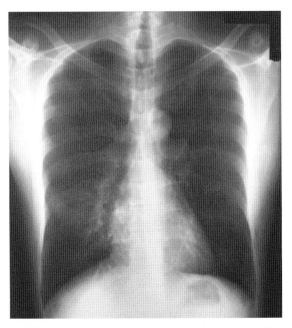

A

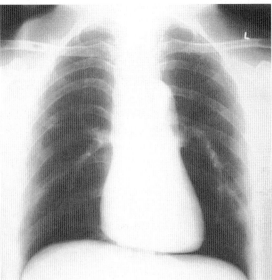

B

Figure 5 Comparison of (A) 100% overexposed (dark) chest radiograph with (B) a properly exposed chest radiograph. (A is reproduced, with permission, from Slone RM, Guitierrez FR, Fisher AJ: *Thoracic Imaging.* McGraw-Hill, New York, 1999; B from Saia DA: *Appleton & Lange's Review for the Radiography Examination,* 4th ed. McGraw-Hill, New York, 2000)

The 15% rule can also be applied to change the penetrating ability of the x-ray beam while maintaining radiographic density. For example, if you want to increase penetration through the heart on a portable chest radiograph, but you want to keep the density the same, you can increase the kV by 15% and halve the mAs on the repeat examination. The repeat radiograph will show increased penetration through the heart, but the over-all density will remain unchanged (Fig. 6). Similarly, if you decrease the kV by 15%, you can double the mAs to maintain the original density. You should understand, however, if you are already using a kV that provides proper penetration, a kV decrease might cause underpenetration of the part. Even though the mAs is doubled, an inadequate amount of energy will pre-vent the x-rays from penetrating the part and reaching the film.

Technical Tip: No amount of mAs can compensate for inadequate kV to obtain the desired density. Therefore, as a general rule, if a radiograph shows adequate penetration of the anatomical parts of interest, the kV setting should not be decreased.

Source-to-Image Receptor Distance (SID)

If the SID must be changed, but you want to maintain a particu-lar density, you must apply the *density maintenance formula* to the original exposure settings. The **density maintenance formula** determines what change in mAs is needed to maintain density after the SID has been changed, and is written as follows:

$$\frac{mAs_1}{mAs_2} = \frac{(SID)_1^2}{(SID)_2^2}$$

➢ *Refer to **Appendix B** for SID Conversion Table*

Grid Conversion Factors

To calculate the new mAs needed when changing grid con-version factors, use the following formula:

$$New\ mAs = Original\ mAs \times \frac{New\ Grid\ Factor}{Old\ Grid\ Factor}$$

➢ *Refer to **Appendix C** for Grid Conversion Factor Table*

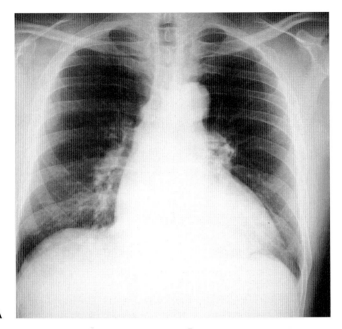

A

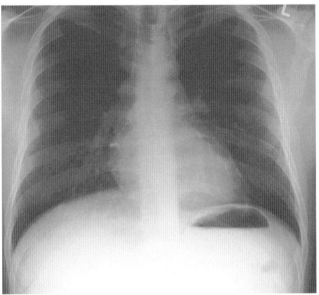

B

Figure 6 Comparison of (A) an underpenetrated chest radiograph with (B) a properly penetrated chest radiograph. The density is similar in both radiographs because the 15% rule requires the mAs to be halved when the kVp is increased by 15%.

Screen–Film Relative Speed

Screen–film combinations are classified according to their **relative speed** (RS). Common relative speed values used in medical imaging departments range from 100 to 400. The following formula can be used to change the mAs when converting from one relative speed to another:

$$\frac{mAs_1}{mAs_2} = \frac{RS_2}{RS_1}$$

➢ *Refer to **Appendix D** for Screen–Film Relative Speed Conversion Table*

Pediatric Radiography

Some pediatric patients require a decrease in exposure factors to compensate for their smaller body parts and less muscle mass as compared to most adult patients.

➢ *Refer to **Appendix E** for Pediatric Conversion Table*

Collimation/Beam Limitation

When using a collimator or extension cylinder to decrease x-ray beam size, the mAs setting must be increased according to how much collimation or beam limitation is applied, based on changes from a 14- × 17-in. (35- × 43-cm) beam size:

- When the beam is collimated from a 14- × 17-in. (35- × 43-cm) beam size to a 10- × 12-in. (25- × 30-cm) beam size, the mAs should be increased by 40%.

- When the beam is collimated from a 14- × 17-in. (35- × 43-cm) beam size to an 8- × 10-in. (20- × 25-cm) beam size, the mAs should be increased by 60%.

- When an extension cylinder is used, and is fully retracted, the mAs should be increased by 40% or 5 kV should be added to the noncylinder exposure technique.

- When the extension cylinder is fully extended, the mAs should be increased by 60% or 10 kV should be added to the noncylinder exposure technique.

Cast Radiography

When radiographing anatomical parts encased in plaster casts, exposure factors must be increased to produce an acceptable radiographic density. The degree of increase depends on whether the plaster cast is *wet* or *dry*.

- When a plaster cast is wet, either add 15 kV or triple the mAs.
- When a plaster cast is dry, either add 10 kV or double the mAs.

  NOTE: To minimize patient dose, it is better to increase kV rather than mAs.

- If only one side of the extremity is covered by a dry plaster splint, add 5 kV.
- If a dry plaster splint curves around the sides of the extremity, the lateral projection will require a 10-kV increase because there are now two sides to penetrate, similar to that experienced when a whole plaster cast is used.

Fiberglass casts generally do not require an increase in technical factors. Some fiberglass casts, however, may cover a plaster splint, and therefore you should inspect the casted extremity carefully to determine what type of cast (or combination of casts) the patient is wearing.

- When a fiberglass cast is very thick (and no plaster splint is present), add 5 kV.

TECHNICAL CONVERSIONS AFFECTING RADIOGRAPHIC CONTRAST

Radiographic contrast is described as either *high contrast* or *low contrast*. Radiographic contrast is the difference in adjacent density shades (or tones) across the radiographic image, and its primary function is to make recorded detail visible. The degree of difference in density between two adjacent structures determines whether an image has high contrast or low contrast. High-contrast images are those containing few gray tones and are mainly black and white, which may also be referred to as *short-scale contrast* images (Fig. 7*A*). Low-contrast images are those containing many gray tones, which may also be referred to as *long-scale contrast* images (Fig. 7*B*). Images with high contrast typically provide enhanced visibility of anatomical detail because the human eye can more readily detect structures when their surrounding structures have significantly different densities (high contrast) than when there are subtle differences in densities (low contrast).

Kilovoltage is the controlling factor of radiographic contrast. The effect of kV on contrast can be summarized as follows:

- High kV = low contrast = long-scale contrast = increased scatter fog = many gray tones
- Low kV = high contrast = short-scale contrast = decreased scatter fog = few gray tones (mostly black and white tones)

> **Technical Tip:** To increase contrast, you can decrease kilovoltage and increase mAs using the 15% rule. To decrease contrast, you can increase kilovoltage and decrease mAs using the 15% rule.

OTHER TECHNICAL CONSIDERATIONS

Pathological Changes

Pathological conditions are classified as either *additive* or *destructive*. **Additive pathology** refers to pathological conditions that alter normal tissue in such a way as to make it hard to penetrate (radiopaque). **Destructive pathology** refers to pathological conditions that alter normal tissue in such a way as to make it easy to penetrate (radiolucent). You should diligently obtain patient history from either the patient's chart or, in the case of an outpatient, from the patient. Of course, many patients do not know they have an underlying pathological condition, but some *are* aware of their condition.

> ➤ *Refer to* ***Appendix F*** *for Pathological Conditions Influencing Radiographic Density*

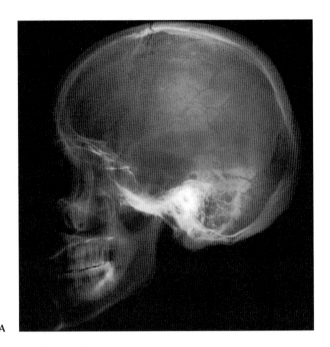

A

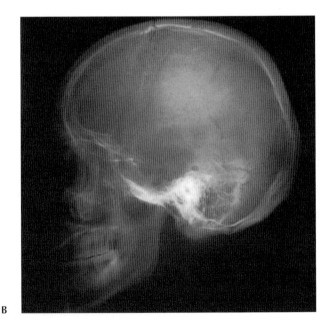

B

Figure 7 Two lateral skull radiographs showing (A) high (short-scale) contrast and (B) low (long-scale) contrast.

44

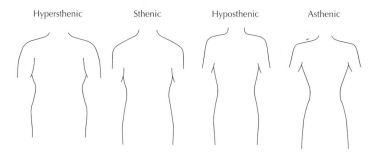

Figure 8 Comparison of various body shapes and sizes.

Body Habitus

The shape and size of the patient is called **body habitus**. The four classifications of body habitus are *hypersthenic, sthenic, hyposthenic,* and *asthenic* (Fig. 8).

- **Hypersthenic habitus** describes a patient having a large body frame.
- **Sthenic habitus** describes an average-sized patient.
- **Hyposthenic habitus** describes a thin patient.
- **Asthenic habitus** describes a thin patient having a very small body frame.

   Of the habitus classifications, hypersthenic habitus patients require the highest exposure settings, and asthenic habitus patients require the lowest exposure settings. The remaining classifications require intermediate exposure settings.

   Thinner parts require less kilovoltage (penetrating power) than do thicker parts. For example, an average size ankle may require a technique of 5 mAs, 60 kV. A thicker ankle may require 5 mAs, 66 kV to produce a similar density.

Technical Tip: A general rule may be applied when the thickness of a part varies up to approximately 5 cm. Simply add or subtract 2 kV for every centimeter of variation from the kV used for a part having average thickness. For parts measuring more than 5 cm thicker or thinner, an accompanying mAs change must also be made.

Image Quality: Photographic Factors

The factors that determine *visibility of detail* on the recorded image are called the **photographic factors**. A proper balance of image density and image contrast is necessary to provide adequate visibility of detail. The radiographer is responsible for determining the exposure settings that will provide this balance. If density and contrast are not optimal, recorded detail cannot be fully appreciated.

> ⮞ *Refer to **Appendix G** for Photographic Factors Affecting Image Quality*

Image Quality: Geometric Factors

Radiography involves the projection of anatomical information onto an image receptor. **Geometric factors** are those factors that affect either *recorded detail* or *distortion*. **Recorded detail** (also called definition, resolution, or sharpness) refers to the fine anatomical structures seen in the recorded image. **Distortion** refers to the inaccurate radiographic representation of either the *size* or *shape* of the anatomical part being radiographed.

> ⮞ *Refer to **Appendix H** for Radiographic Factors and Their Effects on Recorded Detail and Distortion*

Anode Heel Effect

The anode heel effect can be used to an advantage in some radiographic examinations. For body parts that differ in absorption, the anode heel effect can produce radiographs with a more uniform density. For example, in radiography of the thoracic spine, the least intense portion of the beam (anode side) should expose the thinner portion (superior portion). By simultaneously exposing the thicker portion (inferior portion) to the most intense portion of the beam (cathode side), a more uniform density is achieved throughout the image as shown in Figure 9A. If the anode was placed over the thickest portion of the thoracic spine, the superior portion of the spine would be overexposed and the inferior portion of the spine would be underexposed, as shown in Figure 9B.

The anode heel effect is most apparent when using a short SID and a large field size. The following are examples of radiographic examinations for which the anode heel effect may be advantageously used. For each examination listed, the anode side of the beam should be placed over the thinnest portion

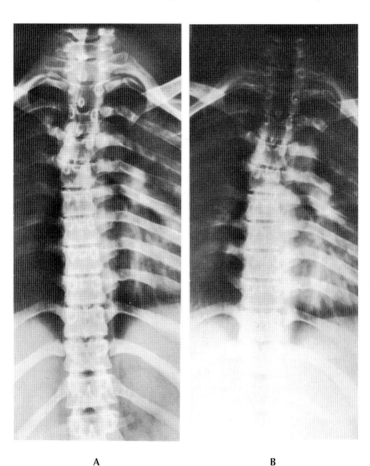

A   B

Figure 9 Two anteroposterior thoracic spine radiographs demonstrating the heel effect. (A) When the x-ray tube is correctly positioned with respect to the thoracic spine, the upper and lower portions of the spine display similar densities. (B) When the x-ray tube is incorrectly positioned, the upper portion of the spine is overexposed and the lower portion of the spine is underexposed. (Courtesy of Eastman Kodak Company)

and the cathode side of the beam should be placed over the thickest portion to improve radiographic density uniformity.

1. AP thoracic spine
2. AP femur
3. AP humerus
4. AP lower leg (tibia/fibula)
5. AP abdomen
6. AP lumbar spine
7. PA chest
8. AP ribs

Technical Tip: The anode end of the x-ray tube is indicated by a positive sign (+), whereas the cathode end of the x-ray tube is indicated by a negative sign (–) marked on the tube housing. If these marks cannot be identified, try boosting the x-ray tube as though you are going to make an exposure. Go into the x-ray room and listen to the x-ray tube at both ends. You can oftentimes hear the anode spinning.

Motion Unsharpness

Motion unsharpness is the most significant form of radiographic unsharpness and appears as either uniform blurring of the entire image of the anatomical part or a specific area of the part, as shown in Figure 10. The exposure time should be kept low when radiographing uncooperative, disoriented, or young pediatric patients to avoid motion unsharpness.

Technical Tip: You can reduce the exposure time and maintain radiographic density by using either of the two following technical changes:

• Increase the mA (if not already using the maximum mA) and decrease the exposure time to provide the desired mAs.

• Use the 15% rule to increase kV and decrease mAs (by decreasing exposure time).

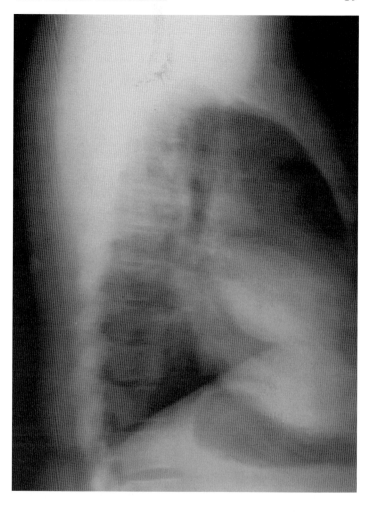

Figure 10 Lateral projection chest radiograph demonstrating motion unsharpness due to patient movement during the exposure.

Autotomography

Sometimes motion unsharpness can be used advantageously, such as in autotomography. When setting a manual technique for autotomography, a low mA setting and a long exposure time is used to allow enough time for blurring of unwanted superimposing structures. For example, if a "breathing tech-

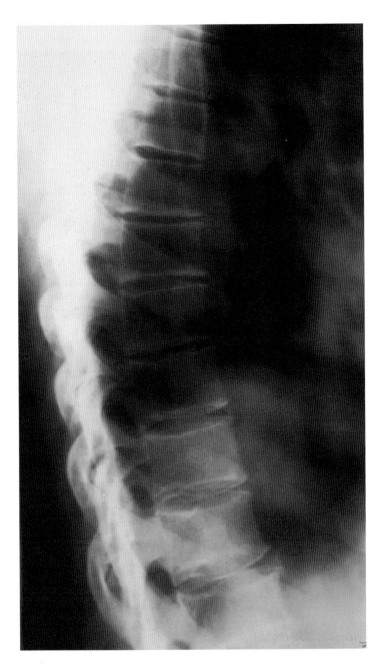

Figure 11 Lateral projection of a thoracic spine using an autotomographic technique. Note how the ribs and vascular structures of the lungs are blurred but the thoracic spine appears sharp.

nique" is used when performing a lateral projection of the thoracic spine, the ribs and the vascular structures of the lungs can be blurred from the image, thus improving visibility as shown in Figure 11.

Technical Tip: When using automatic exposure control (AEC) for a breathing technique, you must use low mA and kV settings and close collimation in order to extend the exposure time long enough to allow for several breathing excursions.

Automatic Exposure Control

Before making a radiographic exposure when using AEC, you should obtain a surgical history from your patient, or from the patient's chart, to rule out the presence of a metal prosthesis. This is particularly important when performing hip or knee radiographic examinations.

Technical Tip: If the anatomical part of interest contains a metal prosthesis, you should use a manual technique rather than AEC.

Magnification

The amount of magnification demonstrated on a radiograph can be determined by calculating the *magnification factor* using the following formulas:

$$MF = \frac{SID}{SOD}$$

or

$$\frac{Image\ Width}{Object\ Width} = \frac{SID}{SOD}$$

You can calculate percent magnification by using the following formula:

$$\% \text{ magnification} = \frac{\text{image width} - \text{object width}}{\text{object width}} \times 100$$

AUTOMATIC EXPOSURE CONTROL: PROBLEMS AND CORRECTIVE ACTIONS

Automatic exposure control allows you to consistently reproduce images having diagnostically acceptable density. When properly used, an *AEC unit* (also called an *automatic exposure device*) will produce consistent density regardless of patient size or pathological condition. Several problems can occur when using AEC, and you must be able to determine the reason and the appropriate corrective action.

> ➢ Refer to **Appendix I** for *Automatic Exposure Control Problems and Corrective Actions*

RADIOGRAPHIC FILM PROCESSING

Processor Factors Causing Excessive Density

- Developer temperature too high
- Developer overreplenishment
- Developer contaminated with fixer
- Processor running too slow
- Developer improperly mixed
- Processor light leak

Processor Factors Causing Insufficient Density

- Developer temperature too low
- Developer underreplenishment; exhausted developer

- Processor running too fast
- Developer improperly mixed

> *Refer to* **Appendix J** *for Developer Components and Their Functions*
> *Refer to* **Appendix K** *for Fixer Components and Their Functions*
> *Refer to* **Appendix L** *for Common Film Artifacts*
> *Refer to* **Appendix M** *for Automatic Processor Maintenance Schedule*

COMPUTED RADIOGRAPHY

Quality control and maintenance is important in computed radiography, just as it is in conventional radiography, to maintain optimum image quality.

NOTE: Any invasive adjustments or corrections should be performed by a qualified vendor technician in cooperation with the department's quality control technologist.

> *Refer to* **Appendix N** *for Computed Radiography Quality Control and Maintenance Schedule*

APPENDIX A

Milliampere-Seconds (mAs) Table

| | | | | | Time in Seconds | | | | | |
mA	0.004 (1/240)	0.008 (1/120)	0.016 (1/60)	0.025 (1/40)	0.033 (1/30)	0.042 (1/24)	0.05 (1/20)	0.067 (1/15)	0.10 (1/10)
50	0.20	0.40	0.80	1.25	1.65	2.1	2.5	3.35	5.0
100	0.40	0.80	1.6	2.5	3.3	4.2	5.0	6.7	10.0
150	0.60	1.2	2.4	3.75	4.95	6.3	7.5	10.05	15.0
200	0.80	1.6	3.2	5.0	6.6	8.4	10.0	13.4	20.0
300	1.2	2.4	4.8	7.5	9.9	12.6	15.0	20.1	30.0
400	1.6	3.2	6.4	10.0	13.2	16.8	20.0	26.8	40.0
500	2.0	4.0	8.0	12.5	16.5	21.0	25.0	33.5	50.0
600	2.4	4.8	9.6	15.0	19.8	25.2	30.0	40.2	60.0
800	3.2	6.4	12.8	20.0	26.4	33.6	40.0	53.6	80.0
1000	4.0	8.0	16.0	25.0	33.0	42.0	50.0	67.0	100

(continued)

Milliampere-Seconds (mAs) Table (Continued)

| | | | | | | | Time in Seconds | | | | | | |
mA	0.125 (1/8)	0.20 (1/5)	0.25 (1/4)	0.30 (3/10)	0.40 (2/5)	0.50 (1/2)	0.60 (3/5)	0.80 (4/5)	1.0
50	6.25	10.0	12.5	15.0	20.0	25.0	30.0	40.0	50.0
100	12.5	20.0	25.0	30.0	40.0	50.0	60.0	80.0	100
150	18.75	30.0	37.5	45.0	60.0	75.0	90.0	120	150
200	25.0	40.0	50.0	60.0	80.0	100	120	160	200
300	37.5	60.0	75.0	90.0	120	150	180	240	300
400	50.0	80.0	100	120	160	200	240	320	400
500	62.5	100	125	150	200	250	300	400	500
600	75.0	120	150	180	240	300	360	480	600
800	100	160	200	240	320	400	480	640	800
1000	125	200	250	300	400	500	600	800	1000

APPENDIX B

The following table can be used as a quick reference to maintain radiographic density when the source-to-image receptor distance (SID) is changed. Simply locate the old SID on the vertical column at left and the new SID on the top horizontal column. Follow horizontally from the old SID to the conversion factor that lies beneath the new SID. Multiply the original mAs by the conversion factor to calculate the new mAs.

Example: If you used 20 mAs at a 40-in. SID, you must multiply 20 mAs by 3.24 if you increased the SID to 72 in. Therefore, 20 mAs × 3.24 = 68.4 (or 65) mAs.

SID Conversion Table

		New SID (in.)				
SID (in.)	*30*	*40*	*50*	*60*	*72*	*120*
30	1.0	1.78	2.78	4.0	5.76	16.0
40	0.56	1.0	1.56	2.25	3.24	9.0
50	0.36	0.64	1.0	1.44	2.07	5.76
60	0.25	0.44	0.69	1.0	1.44	4.0
72	0.17	0.31	0.48	0.69	1.0	2.78
120	0.06	0.11	0.17	0.25	0.36	1.0

Old SID

APPENDIX C

Grid Conversion Factor Table

Grid Ratio	Grid Conversion Factor
No grid	1
5:1	2
6:1	3
8:1	4
12:1	5
16:1	6

APPENDIX D

The following table can be used as a quick reference to maintain radiographic density when the relative speed is changed. Simply locate the old relative speed on the vertical column at the left and the new relative speed on the top horizontal column. Follow horizontally from the old relative speed to the conversion factor that lies beneath the new relative speed. Multiply the original mAs by the conversion factor to calculate the new mAs.

Screen–Film Relative Speed Conversion Table

Relative Screen–Film Speed	New Relative Speed				
	100	200	250	300	400
100	1.0	0.5	0.4	0.33	0.25
200	2.0	1.0	0.8	0.67	0.5
250	2.5	1.25	1.0	0.83	0.63
300	3.0	1.5	1.2	1.0	0.75
400	4.0	2.0	1.6	1.33	1.0

Old Relative Speed

APPENDIX E

Pediatric Conversion Table

Age Group	Age Range	Conversion
Infancy	Birth to 2 y	Multiply mAs by .25
Preschool	2 to 6 y	Multiply mAs by .50
School age	6 to 12 y	Multiply mAs by .75
Teenage	>12 y	No change

APPENDIX F

Pathological Conditions Influencing Radiographic Density

Additive Pathology *(require an increase in kV)*	*Destructive Pathology* *(require a decrease in kV)*
Skeletal system	**Skeletal system**
Proliferative arthritis	Destructive arthritis
Bone callus	Necrosis
Exostosis	Bone cancer (osteolytic)
Hydrocephalus	Osteoporosis
Osteopetrosis	Osteopenia
Osteochondroma	Osteomalacia
Osteoma	Atrophy
Paget's disease	Bone abscess
Acromegaly	
Sclerosis	
Respiratory system	**Respiratory system**
Pneumonia	Emphysema
Pleural effusion	Pneumothorax
Atelectasis	
Bronchiectasis	
Pulmonary edema	
Empyema	
Lung abscess	
Hemothorax	
Hydrothorax	
Pneumoconiosis	
Cardiovascular system	
Cardiomegaly	
Pericardial effusion	
Aneurysm	
Ascites from hepatic cirrhosis	
Gastrointestinal system	**Gastrointestinal system**
Ascites from bowel perforation	Ileus
Soft tissues	**Soft tissues**
Edema	Emaciation
Morbid obesity	

APPENDIX G

Photographic Factors Affecting Image Quality

Factor	Density	Contrast
Increased		
mA	↑	0
Exposure time	↑	0
kV	↑	↓
SID	↓	0
OID	↓	↑
Screen speed	↑	↑
Film speed	↑	↑
Grid factor	↓	↑
Beam restriction	↓	↑
Beam filtration	↓	↓
Collimation	↓	↑
Decreased		
mA	↓	0
Exposure time	↓	0
kV	↓	↑
SID	↑	0
OID	↑	↓
Screen speed	↓	↓
Film speed	↓	↓
Grid factor	↑	↓
Beam restriction	↑	↓
Beam filtration	↑	↑
Collimation	↑	↓

APPENDIX H

Radiographic Factors and Their Effects on Recorded Detail
and Distortion

Factor	Recorded Detail	Distortion
Increased		
mAs	0	0
kV	0	0
SID	↑	↓
OID	↓	↑
Screen speed	↓	0
Film speed	↓	0
Focal spot size	↓	0
Collimation	0	0
CR angle	0	↑
Decreased		
mAs	0	0
kV	0	0
SID	↓	↑
OID	↑	↓
Screen speed	↑	0
Film speed	↑	0
Focal spot size	↑	0
Collimation	0	0
CR angle	0	↓

APPENDIX I

Automatic Exposure Control Problems and Corrective Actions

Problem	Corrective Action Options
Exposure time too long (image displays unwanted motion unsharpness)	1. Increase mA and/or increase kV 2. Decrease SID 3. Check tube/Bucky grid alignment 4. Check image for prosthetic device 5. Check image for additive pathological process
Exposure time too short (causing stroboscopic effect)	1. Decrease mA and/or decrease kV 2. Increase SID
Premature exposure termination (insufficient radiographic density)	1. Check for accurate centering 2. Check detector selection 3. Increase collimation 4. Use lead strip behind patient when performing lateral spine radiography (excluding cervical spine) 5. Increase backup time (when possible). NOTE: Do not allow an exposure that exceeds 600 mAs.
Insufficient radiographic density when using neutral density setting (assuming film processing conditions are optimal)	1. Ensure proper cassette was used 2. Increase density step(s) (+1 = 25% density increase); notify supervisor (equipment should be calibrated)
Excessive radiographic density when using neutral density setting (assuming film processing conditions are optimal)	1. Ensure proper cassette was used 2. Decrease density step(s) (−1 = 25% density decrease); notify supervisor (equipment should be calibrated)
Longer exposure time needed for adequate blurring in autotomography	1. Decrease mA and/or decrease kV 2. Increase SID

APPENDIX J

Developer Components and Their Functions

Component	Chemical Name	Function
Reducing agent	Phenidone	Quickly produces the gray tones in the image
Reducing agent	Hydroquinone	Slowly produces the black tones in the image
Buffering agent	Sodium carbonate	Produces alkaline pH; swells emulsion
Restrainer	Potassium bromide	Antifogging agent; maintains proper reducing agent activity
Preservative	Sodium sulfite	Controls oxidation; provides balance of developer components
Hardener	Gluteraldehyde	Reduces emulsion swelling; hardens emulsion; promotes archival quality
Solvent	Water	Dissolves chemicals

APPENDIX K

Fixer Components and Their Functions

Component	Chemical Name	Function
Fixing agent	Ammonium thiosulfate	Removes undeveloped silver bromide from emulsion
Activator	Acetic acid	Stops development
Hardener	Potassium alum	Hardens emulsion; ensures rapid and complete drying
Preservative	Sodium sulfite	Maintains chemical balance
Buffer	Acetate	Maintains acidic pH
Solvent	Water	Dissolves chemicals

APPENDIX L

Common Film Artifacts

Artifacts running parallel to film travel through automatic processor

Guide shoe marks

Evenly spaced plus-density lines (Fig. 12)

Evenly spaced minus-density lines (Fig. 13A)

Cause

Excessive pressure from misaligned guide shoes

Misalignment of guide shoes; emulsion scratched off base

Entrance roller marks

Plus-density lines (Fig. 14)

Cause

Excessive pressure from entrance rollers or moisture on entrance rollers

Artifacts running perpendicular to film travel through automatic processor

Hesitation marks

Plus-density line(s) usually seen near leading edge of film (Fig. 15)

Cause

Malfunctioning gears or loose chain; warped rollers

Chatter marks

Plus-density lines evenly spaced

Cause

Loose drive gears, chain, or developer-to-fixer crossover-rack assembly

Pi lines

Plus-density lines spaced 3.14 inches apart (Fig. 13B)

Cause

Dirty rollers; emulsion buildup on rollers; developer solution level too low, causing incomplete emersion of top rollers of transport-roller-rack assembly

Random processing artifacts

Water spots

Dull, superficial, and irregular spots or streaks seen best with reflected light

Cause

Malfunctioning squeegee rollers from wash tank; clogged dryer tube(s)

Pick-off

Small, randomly spaced minus-density spots (Fig. 16)

Cause

Rough or dirty rollers lifting small pieces of emulsion off base

Brown tint

Emulsion has brown appearance

Cause

Inadequate film washing

Common Film Artifacts (*Continued*)

Film handling artifacts

Scratches

Linear minus-density marks (Fig. 17)

Cause

Dropping film on floor; sliding film on dirty feed tray; careless insertion of film in film bin or during cassette loading

Static marks

Plus-density marks that may appear randomly across the film (three common types are smudge, crown, and tree static as shown in Fig. 18)

Cause

Low humidity; inadequate grounding of workbench; careless handling of film such as rapidly removing film from cassette or film bin

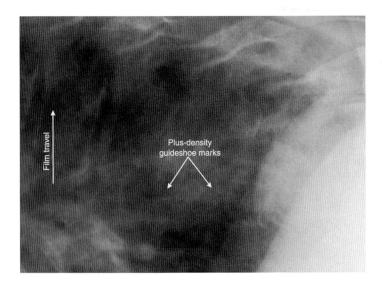

Figure 12 Radiograph showing plus-density guide shoe marks. These artifacts occur when the guide shoes of a radiographic processor become misaligned. In this picture, the linear marks are plus-density due to excessive pressure from the raised ridges of the guide shoes on the radiographically exposed film. Guide shoe marks always run parallel to the film travel direction through the processor.

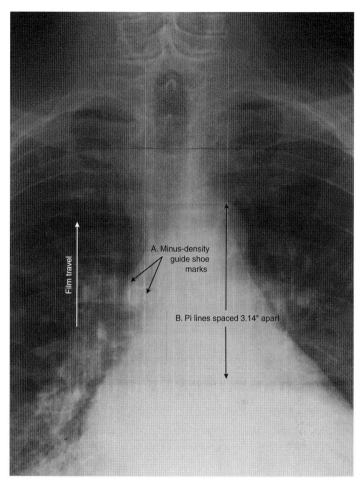

Figure 13 Radiograph demonstrating two processor artifacts. (A) Minus-density guide shoe marks. These artifacts occur when the guide shoes of a radiographic processor become misaligned. In this picture, the linear marks are minus-density due to the removal of emulsion by the raised ridges of the guide shoes on the radiographically exposed film. Guide shoe marks always run parallel to the film travel direction through the processor. (B) Pi lines are seen where deposits from a 1-in. roller are placed 3.14 in. apart on the film. Pi lines always run perpendicular to the film travel direction through the processor.

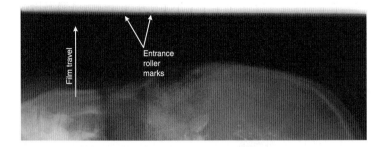

Figure 14 Entrance roller marks caused by excessive entrance roller pressure.

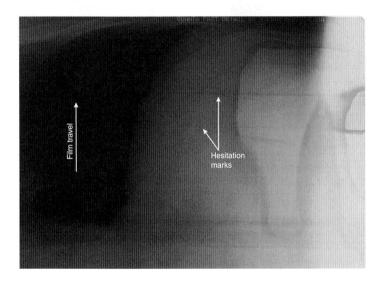

Figure 15 Radiograph demonstrating hesitation marks caused by malfunctioning transport gears or loose drive chains. Warped processor rollers may also produce this artifact.

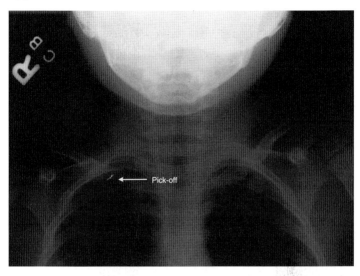

Figure 16 Radiograph demonstrating emulsion pick-off caused by either a rough or dirty processor roller lifting a small piece of the emulsion from the film base.

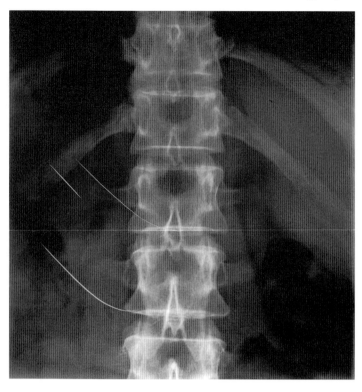

Figure 17 Radiograph demonstrating emulsion scratches. Scratches can occur by dropping the film on the floor, sliding the film on a dirty feed tray, or careless insertion of the film into the film bin or during cassette loading.

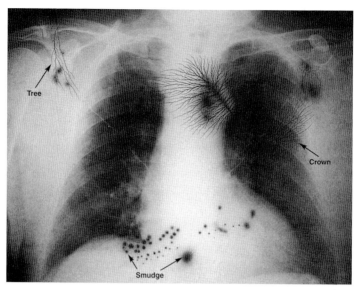

Figure 18 Radiograph demonstrating three common types of static artifacts. These artifacts can occur when the humidity is low, when the darkroom workbench is inadequately grounded, and when film is rapidly removed from the film bin or a cassette. (Reproduced, with permission, from Fosbinder RA, Kelsey CA: Essentials of Radiology Science. McGraw-Hill, 2002)

APPENDIX M

Automatic Processor Maintenance Schedule

Daily	Weekly	Monthly
Wash evaporation covers	Removal, cleaning, and inspection of the transport roller racks; inspection includes checking gears, chains, and rollers for wear and ease of movement	Check alignment of feed tray
Clean crossover racks	Inspect solutions for foreign matter after removing transport roller racks	Check replenishment rates and adjust if needed
Rotate and clean rollers	Turn on circulation pumps and observe solution circulation	Drain and clean all processor tanks
Clean tank deposits above solution level	Inspect all filters	Inspect all tubing and their connections for leaks
Clean deposits from dryer area	Clean dryer air tubes	Lubricate gears according to manufacturer's recommendations
Lift processor lid, leave partially open overnight to vent fumes and reduce chemical condensation on underside of lid	Check replenishment lines for bends, kinks, or debris	Check for proper function of entrance roller microswitch and adjust if needed
		Clean crossover racks and check for any needed repairs

APPENDIX N

Computed Radiography (CR) Quality Control and Maintenance Schedule

Daily

1. Inspect operation of CR scanners, ID terminals, and monitors.
2. Produce laser-generated sensitometry strips and measure optical densities.
3. Check laser processor chemical levels and temperature (if applicable).

Weekly

1. Clean CR system filters.
2. Erase all image plates that are rarely used.
3. Check monitor brightness and contrast settings.
4. Inspect CR cassettes and image plates. Clean as necessary with an ethanol-based cleaner.
5. Acquire quality control test phantom (purchased along with CR system) images and catalog results in computer database; check performance and take corrective action as necessary.

Monthly

1. Perform processor maintenance.
2. Review repeat rates and exposure indices. Determine causes for suboptimal images and exposure inconsistencies.

Annually (Physicist)

1. Perform linearity/sensitivity tests on all image plates.
2. Evaluate image quality; check image processing algorithms.
3. Review repeat rates, patient exposure trends, quality control records, and equipment service history.